Whitman on Wellness

POETRY & PROSE FOR A HEALTHY LIFE

Walt Whitman/Mose Velsor

Edited by Bevin Vieweg-Lenz

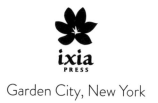

ixia
PRESS

Garden City, New York

Bibliographical Note

This Ixia edition, first published in 2023, is a compilation of excerpts from Walt Whitman's poetry, reprinted from standard editions, along with excerpted articles by Whitman, writing as Mose Velsor, published in *The New York Atlas's* newspaper series *Manly Health and Training with Off-Hand Hints Toward their Conditions* in 1858. Please note that the work presents Velsor's opinions, and his recommendations are not to be regarded as prescriptions for modern-day healthy living.

All images are courtesy of Getty Images.

International Standard Book Number

ISBN-13: 978-0-486-85077-1
ISBN-10: 0-486-85077-3

Ixia Press
An imprint of Dover Publications

Printed in China by Chang Jiang Printing Media Co., Ltd.
85077301   2023
www.doverpublications.com/ixiapress

Introduction

Lauded as the "Bard of Democracy" and one of America's most influential poets, Walt Whitman reveals in his work his lust for life, adoration of nature, and pride for a nation he believed was built on the robust and vital bodies of his fellow Americans. In late editions of *Leaves of Grass*, the wisdom dispersed by the Good Gray Poet reflects unrestrained optimism and loving acceptance for life's evolving seasons, peppered with the understanding that true enjoyment of the many pleasures of living is reliant upon the good health of the body.

Whitman is most recognized for his trademark free verse musings. However, this perception expanded in 2016 when graduate student Zachary Turpin stumbled upon "Manly Health and Training with Off-Hand Hints Toward their Conditions," a series of as yet undiscovered articles written by Whitman in 1858 for *The New York Atlas* under the moniker Mose Velsor, a name he derived from that of his mother, Louisa van Velsor. While it was not unheard-of for Whitman to use a pen name for his journalistic endeavors, the *Manly Health and Training with Off-Hand Hints Toward their Conditions* articles read more like the rantings of a health-obsessed alter ego than merely Whitman hiding behind the curtain of a *nom de plume*. In fact, Velsor is so adamantly convinced that proper training and nutrition are the key to solving all of life's woes that it is hard not to be influenced by his very practical, albeit dogmatic, take on all things wellness (even when served with a side of toxic masculinity).

It might be challenging to reconcile the "live and let live" philosophy that makes Whitman's poetry so accessible with the dictatorial style of Velsor, yet the similarities in syntax and diction are undeniable. Perhaps it is Velsor we can blame for vaingloriously insisting on enhancing the trouser bulge in the frontispiece engraving of the rakish young Whitman that adorns the cover of later printings of *Leaves of Grass*. For this is just the kind of thing one might come to expect after reading all thirteen articles in *The New York Atlas* series. And yet, Mose or Walt, or both, are onto something. Several practices introduced in *Manly Health* are considered fundamental to the current health and fitness zeitgeist, such as dry brushing, cold exposure, nervous system regulation, and even the paleo or "all meat" diet rank among the myriad recommendations for cultivating a "perfect physique."

In an age where, for some, it seems that wellness has taken the place of religion, Whitman's Velsor may have been a sort of prophet in the realm of health and fitness, or at the very least, a self-care influencer (even if such a title didn't yet exist). What follows in these pages is a collection of excerpts from Mose Velsor's 1858 *The New York Atlas* articles paired with some more temperate meditations culled from Whitman's poetry. The intention is to make the sound advice offered in the *Manly Health* articles more palatable. After all, as Velsor will tell you, indigestion is the great American evil.

From **Whoever You Are Holding Me Now in Hand**

Whoever you are holding me now in hand,
Without one thing all will be useless,
I give you fair warning before you attempt me further,
I am not what you supposed, but far different.

Who is he that would become my follower?
Who would sign himself a candidate for my affections . . .

MANLY HEALTH AND TRAINING, WITH OFF-HAND HINTS TOWARD THEIR CONDITIONS

Manly health! Is there not a kind of charm—a fascinating magic in the words? We fancy we see the look with which the phrase is met by many a young man, strong, alert, vigorous, whose mind has always felt but never formed in words, the ambition to attain to the perfection of his bodily powers—has realized to himself that all other goods of existence would hardly be goods, in comparison with a perfect body, perfect blood—no morbid humors, no weakness, no impotency or deficiency or bad stuff in him; but all running over with animation and ardor, all marked by herculean strength, suppleness, a clear complexion, and the rich results (which follow such causes) of a laughing voice, a merry song and night, a sparkling eye, and an ever happy soul!

PRESENT CONDITION OF THE HEALTH
OF THE MASSES

We are not disposed to grumble or overstate the evil condition of the public physique; we wish to call attention to the fact how easily most of these deficiencies might be remedied.

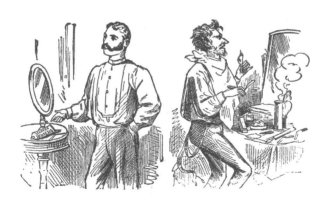

EFFECTS OF A SOUND BODY

Among the signs of manly health and perfect physique, internal and external, are a clear eye, a transparent and perhaps embrowned complexion (this latter not necessarily), an upright attitude, a springy step, a sweet breath, a ringing voice and little or nothing of irritability in the temper.

LIFE WITHOUT A SOUND BODY— WHAT IS IT GOOD FOR?

Reason seems to tell a man, not so much that death is dreadful, as that *dragging out a useless, deficient, and sickly life is dreadful.* We even think that if such a life were to be continued year after year, without probability of change, death would be preferable—would be a happy relief from it.

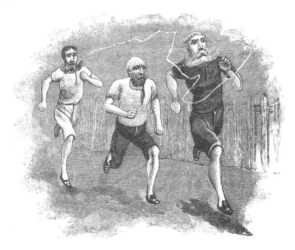

From **I Sing the Body Electric**

... The exquisite realization of health;
O I say these are not the parts and poems of the body only,
    but of the soul,
O I say now these are the soul!

FOR STUDENTS, CLERKS, AND THOSE IN SEDENTARY OR MENTAL EMPLOYMENTS

We say to the young man not only that mental development may well go on at the same time with physical development, but that indeed is the only way in which they should go on—both together, which is much to the advantage of each. If you are a student, be also a student of the body . . . .

Let nothing divert you from your duty to your body. Up in the morning early! Habituate yourself to the brisk walk in the fresh air—to the exercise of pulling the oar—and to the loud declamation upon the hills, or along the shore. Such are the means by which you can seize with treble gripe upon all the puzzles and difficulties of your student life.

To you, clerk, literary man, sedentary person, man of fortune, idler, the same advice. Up! The world (perhaps you now look upon it with pallid and disgusted eyes) is full of zest and beauty for you, if you approach it in the right spirit!

Do not be discouraged soon. Give our advice a thorough trial—not for a few days or weeks, but for months. Early rising, early to bed, exercise, plain food, thorough and persevering continuance in gently-commenced training, the cultivation with resolute will of a cheerful temper, the society of friends and a certain number of hours spent every day in regular employment—these we say, simple as they are, are enough to revolutionize life, and change it from a scene of gloom, feebleness, and irresolution, into *life indeed*, as becomes such a universe as this, full of all the essential means of happiness . . . .

From Song of Myself, 2

Stop this day and night with me and you shall possess the origin
    of all poems,
You shall possess the good of the earth and sun, (there are millions of
    suns left,)
You shall no longer take things at second or third hand, nor look
    through the eyes of the dead, nor feed on the spectres in books,
You shall not look through my eyes either, nor take things from me,
You shall listen to all sides and filter them from your self.

TRAINING

There we print the magic word that can remedy all the troubles and accomplish all the wonders of human physique. Training! In its full sense, it involves the entire science of manly excellence, education, beauty, and vigor—nor is it without intimate bearings upon the moral and intellectual nature.

Training, however, it is always to be borne in mind, does not consist in mere exercise. Equally important with that are the diet, drink, habits, sleep, etc. Bathing, the breathing of good air, and certain other requisites, are also not to be overlooked.

BRIEF SKETCH OF A DAY OF TRAINING, FOR THE USE OF BEGINNERS

The man rises at day-break, or soon after—if in winter, rather before. In most cases the best thing he can commence the day with is a rapid wash of the whole body in cold water, using a sponge, or the hands rubbing the water over the body and then coarse towels to rub dry with; after which, the hair gloves, the flesh-brush, or anything handy, may be used, for friction, and to put skin in a red glow all over. This especially in cool weather, must all be done in a few minutes, or rather moments—not much longer than you have taken to read about it.

This brings us to an early breakfast hour. Usually the breakfast, for a hearty man, might consist in a plate of lean meat, without fat or gravy, a slice or chunk of bread, and, if desired, a cup of tea, which must be left till the last. If there be boiled potatoes, and one of them is desired, it may be permitted. Ham, gravy, fried potatoes, and a list too long and numerous to mention, of dishes often found on the breakfast table of boarding houses and restaurants, must be eschewed.

The great art lies in what to avoid and what to deny one's self.

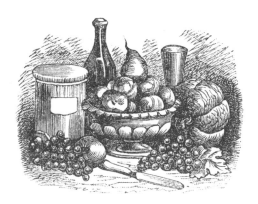

After breakfast, in the case of a man who has work to do, (for we are writing for the general public, as well as the sporting man,) he will go about his employment. One who has not, and who is devoting his attention, at the time, to the establishment of health and a manly physique, will do well to spend an hour of the forenoon (say from 10 to 11 o'clock,) in some good exercise for the arms, hands, breast, spine, shoulders, and waist; the dumb-bells, sparring, or a vigorous attack on the sand-bags, (a large bag, filled with sand, and suspended in such a position that it can be conveniently struck with the fists). This should be done systematically, and gradually increased upon making the exertion harder and harder.

A pretty long walk may also be taken, commencing at an ordinary pace, and increasing the rapidity of the step till it takes the power of locomotion pretty well, and then keeping it up at that gait, as it can be well endured—not to the extent of fatigue, however, for it is a law of training that *a man must not exercise so hard as to overdo and tire himself*; but always stop in time to avoid fatigue.

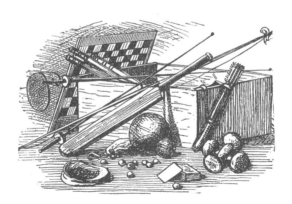

From three quarters to half an hour before dinner, all violent exercise must cease.

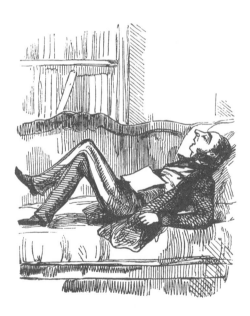

If the body is sweaty, as it very likely will be, it is best to strip, rub down briskly with dry cloths, and change the underclothes.

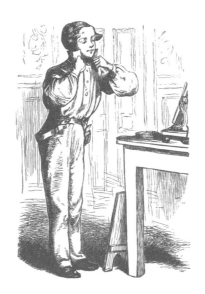

Dinner should consist of a good plate of fresh meat, (rare lean beef, broiled or roast, is best) with as few outside condiments as possible. (If thirsty during the forenoon, drink, but never before eating.) Eat according to your appetite, of one dish always, if possible, making four or five dinners out of the week, of rare lean beef, with nothing else than a small slice of stale bread.

No scraggly, grisly fat, or hard cooked pieces, should be eaten. Nor need the appetite be stinted—eat enough, and when you eat that, stop!

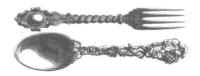

No man should be required to do any toilsome work or exercise immediately after dinner; if there be anything you know you will have to take hold of immediately, then make the dinner lighter, for it is more hurtful than is supposed, to exert one's physical powers greatly, on a hearty meal.

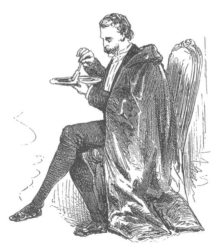

We have thus indicated the mode of filling up the hours of the day; but still more is necessary. After a moderate supper, of some digestible dish, fruit, or cold meat, or stale bread, toast, or biscuit, with perhaps a cup of tea the evening ought to be devoted, to some extent at least, to friendly and social recreation, (not dissipation, remember). Friends may be visited, or some amusement, or a stroll in company or any other means that will soothe and gratify the mind and the affections, friendship, etc., for every man should pride himself on *having* such affections, and satisfying them, too.

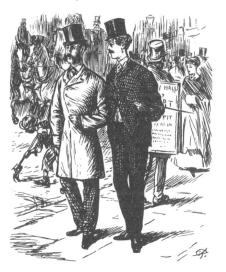

Ten o'clock at night ought to find a man in bed—for that will not afford him the time requisite for rest, if he rise betimes in the morning. The bedroom must not be small and close—that would go far toward spoiling all other observances and cares for health. It is important that the system should be clarified, through the inspiration and respiration, with a plentiful supply of good air, during the six, seven, or eight hours that are spent in sleep. During most of the year, the window must be kept partly open for this purpose.

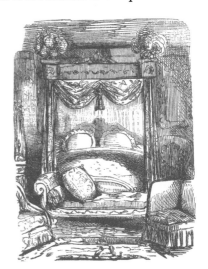

From **When I Heard at the Close of Day**

... But the day when I rose at dawn from the bed of perfect health,
　　refresh'd, singing, inhaling the ripe breath of autumn,
When I saw the full moon in the west grow pale and disappear in the
　　morning light,
When I wander'd alone over the beach, and undressing bathed,
　　laughing with the cool waters, and saw the sun rise,
And when I thought how my dear friend my lover was on his way
　　coming, O then I was happy,
O then each breath tasted sweeter, and all that day my food nourish'd
　　me more, and the beautiful day pass'd well, And the next came with
　　equal joy, ...

EARLY RISING

The habit of rising early is not only of priceless value in itself, as a means toward, and concomitant of health, but is of equal importance from what the habit carries with it, apart from itself.

It is worth noting that the law of rising early necessitates the habit of retiring to bed in good season, which cuts off many of the dissipations most injurious in their effects upon the health. So important is this, that he who should adopt this rule alone will go a great way toward a complete reform—if reform be needed.

A gentle and moderate refreshment at night is admissible enough; and, indeed, if accompanied with the convivial pleasure of friends, the cheerful song, or the excitement of company, and the wholesome stimulus of surrounding good fellowship, is every way to be commended.

From Song of Myself, 2

The smoke of my own breath,
Echoes, ripples, buzz'd whispers, love-root, silk-thread, crotch
    and vine,
My respiration and inspiration, the beating of my heart, the passing of
    blood and air through my lungs,
The sniff of green leaves and dry leaves, and of the shore and dark-
    color'd sea-rocks, and of hay in the barn,
The sound of the belch'd words of my voice loos'd to the eddies of
    the wind,
A few light kisses, a few embraces, a reaching around of arms,
The play of shine and shade on the trees as the supple boughs wag,
The delight alone or in the rush of the streets, or along the fields and
    hill-sides,
The feeling of health, the full-noon trill, the song of me rising from
    bed and meeting the sun.

OUT-DOORS

In that word is the great antiseptic—the true medicine of humanity…. Few know what virtue there is in the open air. Beyond all charms or medications, it is what renews vitality, and, as much as the nightly sleep, keeps the system from wearing out and stagnating upon itself.

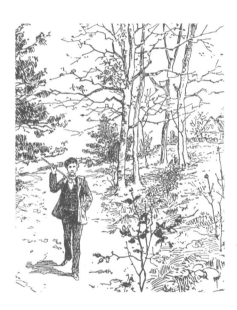

From **When I Heard the Learn'd Astronomer**

. . . How soon unaccountable I became tired and sick,
Till rising and gliding out I wander'd off by myself,
In the mystical moist night-air, and from time to time,
Look'd up in perfect silence at the stars.

MORAL RESULTS OF TRAINING

The results of properly chosen and well-continued courses of training are so valuable and so numerous that in mentioning them we would seem to be mentioning most of the precious treasures of character— among the rest may be specified courage, quickness of all the perceptions, full use of power, independence, fortitude, good nature, a hopeful and sunny temper, an industrious disposition, temperance in all the alimentative appetites, chastity, an aversion to artificial indulgences, easy manner without affectation, personal magnetism, and a certain silent eloquence of expression, and a general tendency to the wholesome virtues and to that moral uprightness which arises out of and is the counterpart of the physical.

MENTALITY, STUDY, ETC., IN THEIR RELATIONS TO HEALTH

Let it be known that a certain degree of abandon is necessary to the processes of perfect health and a muscular tone of the system. The fault of intellectual persons is, doubtless, not only that far too much of their general, natural fund of stimulation is diverted, year after year, from all the great organs in the trunk of the body, and concentrated in the brain, but that they think too much of health, and, perhaps, that they know too much of its laws. Of this last, it might be explained that if they only knew a little more, namely, to put their technical knowledge aside at times, and not be forever dwelling upon it, things would go on much better with them.

From One's-Self I Sing

. . . Of physiology from top to toe I sing,
Not physiognomy alone nor brain alone is worthy for the Muse,
  I say the Form complete is worthier far,
The Female equally with the Male I sing.

WHO CAN FOLLOW THESE RULES?

We are well aware that, to those unaccustomed to consider the laws of health and a sound physique, there will appear at first something quite alarming and impracticable in these requirements. But they are really more so in appearance, and from their novelty, than anything else.

Besides, we are willing to admit that our exact statements with regard to diet—what must be avoided, and the few simple articles of food that, coincident with exercise, strength, digestion, etc., may be used— are to be often modified to suit cases, tastes, etc., each one for itself. We have made the statement of a model case; if the reader approaches the neighborhood of it, he will be doing well.

WE DO NOT INCULCATE A MERE PASTIME

Of exercise, games, gymnastics, etc., the reader must understand well that we inculcate the regular and appropriate practicing of them not as a frivolous pastime, or a matter of ceremony and politeness, to be done in a genteel club way but as *a real living thing, a part of a robust and perfect man.*

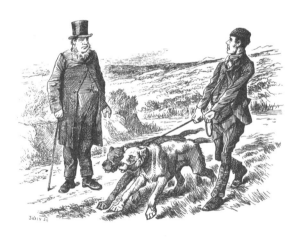

We say *conscientiously*, and we mean all that is involved in the word. The man must himself feel the importance of the objects to be attained, and an enthusiastic, yet in a certain sense calm determination to strive for them not for a little while merely, but for a long while, at work or play, in company or alone, in one place or another, and night and day. *Habit* will soon make all easy; and let us inform you, reader, there is no small pleasure in the victory one attains, by a little sternness of will, over all the deleterious gratification of appetite. It is as great as a general gaining an important battle.

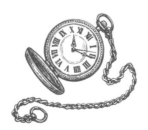

From **The House of Friends**

Fight on, band braver than warriors,
Faithful and few as Spartans;
But fear not most the angriest, loudest malice—
Fear most the still and forked fang
That starts from the grass at your feet.

REGULAR OCCUPATION

A steady and agreeable occupation is one of the most potent adjuncts and favorers of health and long life. The idler, without object, without definite direction, is very apt to brood himself into some moral or physical fever—and one is about as bad as the other.

Disappointment, love, business troubles, and a long list of dark possibilities, are always waiting around every man; these interact, when they happen, (and none can go through life without them) in many ways upon the health. When they do happen, it is no excuse for "giving up"; if one will only persevere in the wholesome observances, and patiently wait a few days, the mind will be again at ease, and spring up with cheerful vigor again.

From O Me! O Life!

The question, O me! so sad, recurring—What good amid these,
    O me, O life?

Answer
That you are here—that life exists and identity,
That the powerful play goes on, and you may contribute a verse.

BACKSLIDING FROM HEALTHY HABITS

After a shorter or longer time, it is quite certain to us there will be
a relapse, however, into the old and more careless ways. A great
revolution, a new system of physical habits, cannot be inaugurated
quite so easily as you thought. Consequently, with the best intentions
in the world, there is still lamentable backsliding. . . . But the work
must not be given up for the first failure—nor even for the second,
third, nor any number. It will gradually grow easier and easier, and
habit will then make it followed, without thinking anything about it.

It must be realized, throughout, that perpetual care is indispensable
to health. It is just as reasonable to suppose you can squander your
fortune at random, and still find it remaining at the end of many years,
as that you can squander your health and have that remain.

OVERTASKING

We must dwell a moment specially here. Let it not be supposed that this question of exercise presents but one side, and that evil to the general health comes from not enough activity. Much is to be said also of the injury of casually overtasking the frame, as is done by many persons, and often at the very times of life when the injury is most fatal to the future soundness and perfection of the body—we mean youth and early manhood.

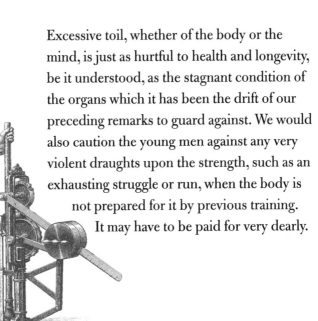

Excessive toil, whether of the body or the mind, is just as hurtful to health and longevity, be it understood, as the stagnant condition of the organs which it has been the drift of our preceding remarks to guard against. We would also caution the young men against any very violent draughts upon the strength, such as an exhausting struggle or run, when the body is not prepared for it by previous training.

It may have to be paid for very dearly.

From **Song of Myself, 1 & 5**

I loafe and invite my soul,
I lean and loafe at my ease observing a spear of summer grass . . .

Loafe with me on the grass, loose the stop from your throat,
Not words, not music or rhyme I want, not custom or lecture,
    not even the best,
Only the lull I like, the hum of your valvèd voice.

NOT TOO VIOLENT EXERCISE

The great object is to have the body in a condition of strong equilibrium—but very violent exertions defeat this end.

❖ ❖ ❖

The fund of vigor and stamina must be used constantly, and encouraged to develope itself gently, but never violently abused.

❖ ❖ ❖

In training exercises, as before remarked, begin and keep on for a few days with great moderation. "Gently does it," is the motto which must never be forgotten. The custom among some young men of trying to perform very difficult and dangerous feats should be discouraged.

From Come Up from the Fields Father

Above all, lo, the sky so calm, so transparent after the rain, and with
  wondrous clouds,
Below too, all calm, all vital and beautiful, and the farm prospers well.

VIRILITY

A man that exhausts himself continually among women, is not fit to be, and cannot be, the father of sound and manly children. They will be puny and scrofulous—a torment to themselves and to those who have the charge of them.

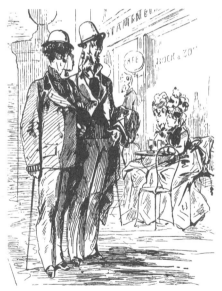

BIRTH-INFLUENCES—BREEDING SUPERB MEN

It is a profound reflection, deeply intertwined with our subject, that much of a man's comfort or discomfort, body and mind, depends on causes that exist and operate, in full activity, before his birth . . . . Unfortunately, however, there has never yet been found a generation that would shape its course, or give up any of its pleasures, for the greater perfection of the generation which was to follow.

No considerations of morbid modesty should be allowed to stand in the way; and, indeed, are not those the immodest ones who would prohibit the enlightenment of the world, both men and women, grown and ungrown, upon what is so vital to them, and to all who come after them . . . .

THE MAGNETIC ATTRACTION FROM HEALTH AND A MANLY PHYSIQUE—CAN IT BE ATTAINED BY TRAINING?

What is it at the bottom of the curious magnetism such men possess, and show it in house or street, in command, in the lecture-room, in the social circle, in politics, or on the field of battle? It is the subtle virtue of their physique—this just as much as intellect.

A man of large personality, (it is not a matter of physical size—a small man may have it as well as any one,) is probably one of the most interesting studies in the world, and one of the greatest exemplifications of our theory of man's vigor. There he is, an evidence of power, of health, of tone—registering all in his port, his carriage, the atmosphere of influence that effuses out of him whenever he moves.

Then observe our suggestions—train—acquire for yourself firm fibres, a stomach clear and capable, the brain-action unabused, the stream of vital power full and voluminous, a bright eye, a strong voice, a proper degree of flesh, a transparent complexion—a fine average yet plus condition; and sympathy, attraction, and a heroic presence will follow. Are these trifles? Not a bit of it.

To all, however, it is a great power—an art well worth the cultivation. Indeed, in the movements of common life, in the usual residence, and in company of acquaintances and friends—there we should say would be found its most grateful spheres of operation—for there the happiness of life, in the man, must rest.

From I Sing the Body Electric

I have perceiv'd that to be with those I like is enough,
To stop in company with the rest at evening is enough,
To be surrounded by beautiful, curious, breathing, laughing flesh is
    enough,
To pass among them or touch any one, or rest my arm ever so lightly
round his or her neck for a moment, what is this then?
I do not ask any more delight, I swim in it as in a sea.

SWIMMING AND BATHING

Many advantages are here concentrated in one—for swimming, being relieved of all the clothes, and supported in the water, allows of bringing nearly all the muscles of the body into easy and pleasant action. Persons habituated to a daily summer swim, or to the rapid wash with cold water over the whole body in the water, are far less liable to sudden colds, inflammatory diseases, or to the suffering of chronic complaints…. It is probably one of the most ancient of health-generating and body-perfecting exercises.

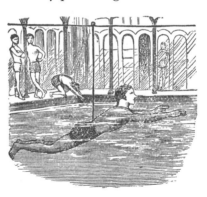

TOO MUCH BRAIN ACTION AND FRETTING

The intellect is too restless. The parent bequeaths the tendency to the child—and he, when grown up, has it in increased force. Some direct it toward money-making, others to religion, and so on. It eats into the whole temperament, and produces reaction; then for fits of "the blues," and an unhappy life.

The remedy lies with the person himself. He must let up on his brain and thought-power, and form more salutary and reasonable habits—which by-the-way, are formed astonishingly soon, if once sternly resolved upon, and the practice commenced in earnest. The homely advice to "take things easy," applies with particular force to this sort of person.

Most of the ills they labor under, and the dispensations they dread, are imaginary; at any rate, imagination distorts them, and magnifies them out of all proportion. A little calmness and coolness puts to flight three-fourths of the evils of their lives.

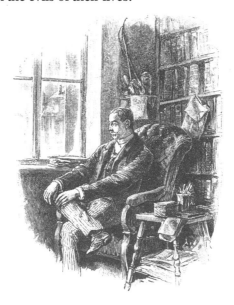

From the Preface to **Leaves of Grass**

This is what you shall do: Love the earth and sun and the animals, despise riches, give alms to everyone that asks, stand up for the stupid and crazy, devote your income and labor to others, hate tyrants, argue not concerning God, have patience and indulgence toward the people, take off your hat to nothing known or unknown, or to any man or number of men, go freely with powerful uneducated persons, and with the young, and with the mothers of families, re-examine all you have been told in school or church or in any book, and dismiss whatever insults your own soul, and your very flesh shall be a great poem, and have the richest fluency, not only in its words, but in the silent lines of its lips and face, and between the lashes of your eyes, and in every motion and joint of your body.

"LOATHED MELANCHOLY" ... THE ONLY RADICAL CURE

It is at least probable, we begin by saying, that in a vast majority of cases, melancholy of mind is the exclusive result of a disordered state of the body—a longer or shorter absence of those clarifying habits of diet exercise, etc.

If the victim of "the horrors" could but pluck up energy enough, after turning the key of his door-lock, to strip off all his clothes and give his whole body a stinging rub-down with a flesh-brush till the skin becomes all red and aglow—then, donning his clothes again, take a long and brisk walk in the open air, expanding the chest and inhaling plentiful supplies of the health-giving element—ten to one but he would be thoroughly cured of his depression, by this alone.

What does this too prevailing melancholy in such people result from? From their bad condition of body, very generally—the reaction of the powers, often from the stimulus of drink, or other exciting causes. In those that do not drink, the stomach and nervous system are very likely out of order, after months, perhaps years, of heedless violations of natural laws.

For this same curse of sadness, in its numberless forms, is an attribute of civilized life, and must be met with those weapons which can destroy it—an infusion through civilized life of a greater degree of natural physical habits, and a stern rejection of those specious enjoyments that leave such frightful deposits afterward, that sting and fester through the middle and later years.

Nor let any one be deceived in this matter of low spirits, by the outside appearance of people as they move about in the streets, in public houses, places of amusement, etc. In public, no doubt you would judge from the show upon the surface that every one was happy, and that there was no such thing as a cloud upon the sky of the mind; all goes so well, and there is so much drinking and eating, and joking and laughing and gay music. The faces are full of color, the eyes sparkle, the voices have a ring—everybody is well dressed, and there is surely no unhappiness in these lives. A serious mistake!

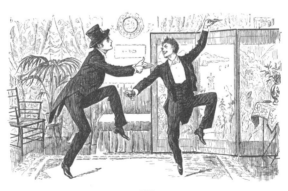

From To You

There is no endowment in man or woman that is not tallied in you,
There is no virtue, no beauty in man or woman, but as good is in you,
No pluck, no endurance in others, but as good is in you,
No pleasure waiting for others, but an equal pleasure waits for you.

STUDY OF THEORIES OF HEALTH

One of the greatest mistakes made in arbitrary theories of certain things supposed to be conducive to health, is that they forget that the true theory of health is multiform, and does not consist of one or two rules alone. The vegetarian, for instance, insists on the total salvation of the human race, if they would only abstain from animal food! This is ridiculous. Others have their hobbies—some of one kind, some of a different. But it is often to be noticed that, in the same person, habits exist that mutually contradict each other, and are parts of opposite theories.

A system of health, in order to be worth following, ought to be consistent in all its parts, and complete besides; and then followed faithfully for a long time .... It is also to be understood that every man's case requires something specially applicable to it.

From **Song of Myself, 51**

Do I contradict myself?
Very well then I contradict myself,
(I am large, I contain multitudes.)

HEALTH OR DISEASE FOLLOW REGULAR LAWS

It is too generally taken for granted that the formation and preservation of manly strength, and of all those points that conduce to longevity, are the result of accidents, haphazard chances, "luck." We wish distinctly to impress it upon the reader that, speaking in general terms, there is no haphazard or luck about the matter.

We repeat it, health and manly strength are under the control of regular and simple laws, and will surely follow the adoption of the means which we have jotted down in the foregoing articles.

BAD BLOOD

In the shortest way of stating it the cause of disease is bad blood—often hereditary, more often from persistence in bad habits. The object of training is, it may also be stated, to simply purify and invigorate the blood—and when that result is attained, to keep it so.

❖ ❖ ❖

Certain habits, be it definitely understood, invariably produce bad blood and a lowered tone of the system—if continued long enough, ending in what is generally called "a ruined constitution."

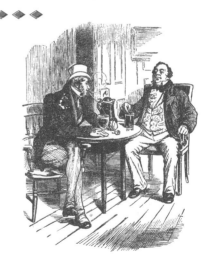

There is, (to make a primitive statement of the matter,) always so much latent possibility of disease in a man's body—as it were sleeping there, ready to be waked up at any time into powerful and destructive action. So long as the system is kept in good order by healthy observances, there is no trouble from these latent germs; but all forms of dissipation and violations of natural law arouse them and cause them to come rapidly forward.

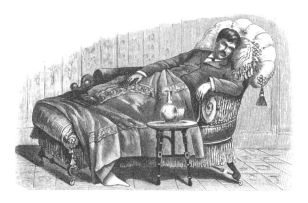

MEDICINES—DO THEY DO ANY GOOD?

We are clear in our own mind that, in by far the vast majority of cases, these medicines do a great deal more hurt than good—that, indeed, they often lay the foundation for a permanent derangement of health, destroy comfort, and shorten life. These are severe words, but we believe them fully warranted by the facts.

The cure must be by other means, and nature, as in all else, is to be looked to, studied, followed, and faithfully relied upon. In general terms it may be stated that the cure must be as slow as the disease was in forming.

BEAUTY

Beauty is simply health and a sound physique. We can hardly conceive of a man, at any age of life, who is in perfect health, and keeps his person clean and neatly attired, who has not some claims to this much-prized attribute.

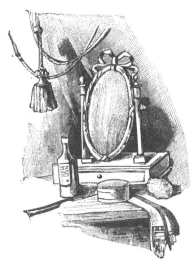

THE SENSES

Indeed, all the senses, all the functions and attributes of the body, become altogether renewed, more refined, more capable of conferring pleasure in themselves, with far more delicate susceptibilities, under the condition produced by long and faithful observance of good diet, proper exercise, and the other rules of healthy development.

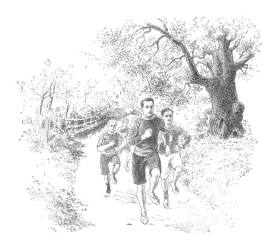

VIRTUE OF OUT-DOORS, AND A STIRRING LIFE

Often, a complete change of scene, associations, companionship, habits, etc., is the best thing that can be done for a man's health, (and the change is perhaps beneficial to a further extent in his morals, knowledge, etc.). If you are "in a bad way" from associations, etc., wisdom and courage both indicate to you to pull up stakes and leave for a new spot—careful there to begin aright, and persevere with energy.

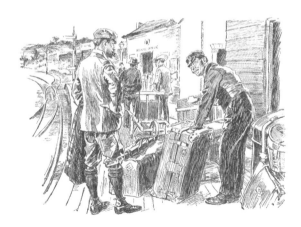

From **Miracles**

To me, every hour of the light and dark is a miracle,
Every cubic inch of space is a miracle,
Every square yard of the surface of the earth is spread with the same,
Every foot of the interior swarms with the same;
Every spear of grass—the frames, limbs, organs, of men and women,
    and all that concerns them,
All these to me are unspeakably perfect miracles.

THE FEET

If a man wants personal ease, and even for health we consider it requisite too, he must pay more than the usual attention to the feet, and what is worn upon them.

It is a singular fact that what might be supposed such a simple accomplishment as perfect and graceful walking, is very rare—is hardly ever seen in the streets of our cities. We have plenty of teachers of dancing—yet to walk well is more desirable than the finest dancing.

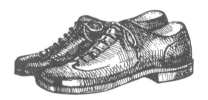

In one of the feet there are thirty-six bones, and the same number of joints, continually playing in locomotion, and needing always a free and loose action. Yet they are always squeezed into boots not modeled from them, nor allowing the play and ease they require .... Probably there is no way to have good and easy boots or shoes, except to have lasts modeled exactly to the shape of the feet. This is well worth doing.

The feet, too, must be kept well clothed with thin socks in summer, and woolen in winter—and washed daily. We may mention that one of the best remedies for cold feet which many people are troubled with in the winter, is bathing them frequently in cold water. If this does not succeed, add a little exercise.

THE THROAT

The beard is a great sanitary protection to the throat—for purposes of health it should always be worn, just as much as the hair of the head should be.

◆ ◆ ◆

Of the throat, it may, perhaps, as well be added that its health and strength are doubtless aided by forming the habit of throwing the voice out from it, and not from the mouth only, as many do.

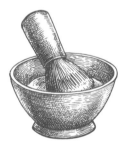

TRAINING THE VOICE

This should be systematic and daily; it strengthens and develops all the large organs, opens the chest, and not only gives decision and vigor to the utterance, in common life, and for all practical purposes, but has a most salutary effect on the throat, with its curious and exquisite machinery, hardening it all, and making it less liable to disease.

We would recommend every young man to select a few favorite poetical or other passages, of an animated description, and get in the habit of declaiming them, on all convenient occasions—especially when out upon the water, or by the sea-shore, or rambling over the hills on the country. Let him not be too timid or bashful about this, but throw himself into it with a will.

From **Song of Myself, 52**

I too am not a bit tamed, I too am untranslatable,
I sound my barbaric yawp over the roofs of the world.

DRINK

We think that water, tea, coffee, soda, lemonade, "slops" of all sorts, have also produced, and are producing, immense injury to the health of the people—from their being used in too great quantities and at wrong times.

We are fain to say, also, that very much of the violent crusade of modern times against brewed and distilled liquors is far from being warranted by the true theory of health, and of physiological laws, as long as those liquors are not partaken of in improper quantities and at injudicious times, disturbing the digestion. Of the two, indeed, we would rather, a little while after his dinner, a man should drink a glass of good ale or wine than one of those mixtures called "soda," or even a strong cup of hot coffee.

MORE ABOUT EATING AND DRINKING

Have greater care, very much greater care, in the choice of articles used for your food, and also in the manner of their being cooked.

What then may be eaten? If you want to know what is best to a hearty man, who takes plenty of exercise and fresh air, and don't want any pimples on his face or body, we will answer, (perhaps very much to your astonishment,) a simple diet of rare-cooked beef, seasoned with a little salt, and accompanied with stale bread or sea-biscuit. Mutton, if lean and tender, is also commendable. Pork should not be eaten.

Butter, pepper, catsup, oil, and most of the "dressings," must also be eschewed . . . there is no sauce like regular and daily exercise, and fresh air.

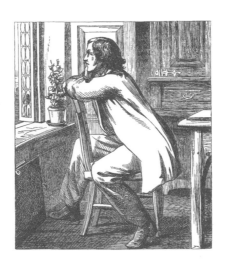

Salted meats are not to be partaken of either; and salt itself, as a seasoning, is to be used as sparingly as possible.

◆ ◆ ◆

With early rising and "taking an airing," there will be no need of an appetite for breakfast, which, under the rules we have stated, may be pretty fully indulged in.

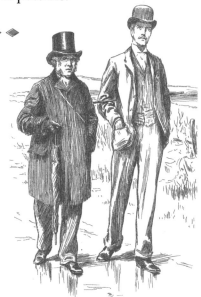

Among the additional rules that may be mentioned with regard to eating, are such as follow:

Make the principal part of your meal always of one dish.

Chew the food well, and do not eat fast.

Wait until you feel a good appetite before eating—even if the regular hour for a meal has arrived.

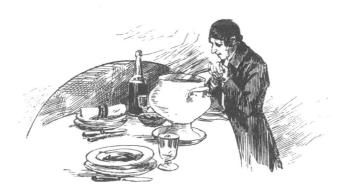

We have spoken against the use of the potato. It still remains to be said that if it agrees with you, and you are fond of it, it may be used; it is best properly boiled, at the morning meal.

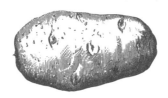

Drink very sparingly at each meal; better still not at all—only between meals, when thirsty.

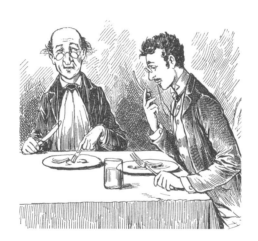

VEGETABLE DIET

We neither practice the vegetarian system ourselves, nor do we recommend it to others as anything like what its enthusiastic advocates claim it to be; and yet we think vegetarianism well worth a respectful mention.

Nearly all of the early philosophers and saints appear to have been men who observed this diet; and, it must also be said, nearly all of them obtained a very advanced period of life . . . . It gives a lustre, a spiritual intelligence to the countenance, that has something saint-like and divine.

This is, of course, a little enthusiastic. We have seen New England and New York vegetarians, gaunt, hard, melancholy, and unhappy looking persons, that looked like anything else than a recommendation of their doctrine—for that is the proof, after all.

From This Compost

. . . The grass of spring covers the prairies,
The bean bursts noiselessly through the mould in the garden,
The delicate spear of the onion pierces upward,
The apple-buds cluster together on the apple-branches,
The resurrection of the wheat appears with pale visage
   out of its graves.
What chemistry!

MEAT AS THE PRINCIPAL DIET FOR THE INHABITANTS OF THE NORTHERN STATES

In our view, if nine-tenths of all the various culinary preparations and combinations, vegetables, pastry, soups, stews, sweets, baked dishes, salads, things fried in grease, and all the vast array of confections, creams, pies, jellies, etc., were utterly swept aside from the habitual eating of the people, and a simple meat diet substituted in their place—we will be candid about it, and say in plain words, an almost exclusive meat diet—the result would be greatly, very greatly, in favor of that noble-bodied, pure-blooded, and superior race we have had a leaning toward, in these articles of ours.

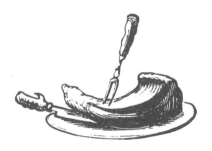

THE GREAT AMERICAN EVIL—INDIGESTION

There can be no good health, or manly and muscular vigor to the system, without thorough and regular digestion . . . . All other rules and requisites may be attended to, but if the stomach be out of order, and allowed to remain so for any length of time, all will be of no avail. We are fain to alter one of the stereotyped sayings of the politicians, and say, Eternal vigilance is the price of—digestion!

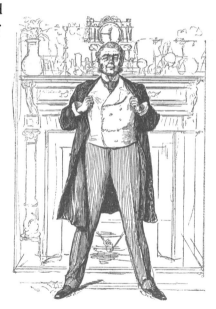

We say to you, reader, do justice to the peculiarities of your own case, with regard to your particular wants, strength, age, trade, previous and present circumstances, etc.; always having in view the main object, regular digestion.

Do not depend on medicines to place your stomach in order; that is but casting out devils through Beelzebub, the prince of devils.

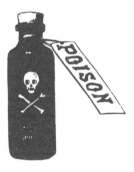

NIGHT-EATING

Portions of heavy food, or large quantities of any kind, taken at evening, or any time during the night, attract an undue amount of the nervous energy to the stomach, and give an overaction to the feelings and powers, which is sure to be followed the next day by more or less bad reactionary consequences; and, if persevered in, must be a strong constitution indeed which does not break down.

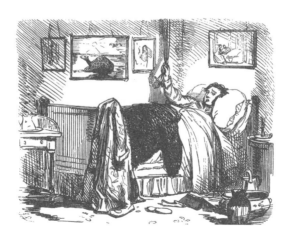

Somebody has said that "we dig our graves with our teeth." There is a great deal of exaggerated statement about the evils of hearty eating, (we mean of plain food)—but it is very true that this habit we are complaining of, and endeavoring to guard the reader against, *habitual night-eating*, quite justifies the proverb.

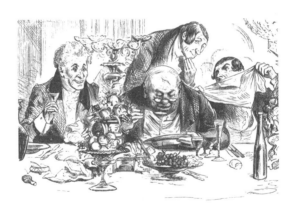

CLIMATE—IS THIS OF OURS CONSISTENT WITH LONGEVITY AND PERFECT HEALTH?

Indeed it seems as if some of the most rugged and unfavorable climates turn out the noblest specimens of men ... for that, among the rest, awakes them to exertion, labor, knowledge, and ingenuity, which develop the great qualities of a man.

❖ ❖ ❖

The cold bath, for instance, cautiously begun, and kept up habitually morning after morning, year after year—what a toughener and hardener to this changeable climate of ours it is!

❖ ❖ ❖

It does not seem to be known that the best way to keep really warm in winter, (for men,) is, not to withdraw from the open air, but go out in it, and keep stirring. Habit soon settles the matter.

From **Song of Myself, 14**

I am enamour'd of growing out-doors,
Of men that live among cattle or taste of the ocean or woods,
Of the builders and steerers of ships and the wielders of axes and
    mauls, and the drivers of horses,
I can eat and sleep with them week in and week out.